Cocaine Treatment: A Guide

Arnold M. Washton, Ph.D.
and Mark S. Gold, M.D.

Copyright © 1986 The American Council for Drug Education
Library of Congress Catalog Card Number: 86-071855

ISBN: 942348-18-4

About the Authors

ARNOLD M. WASHTON, Ph.D.

Arnold M. Washton, Ph.D. is Executive Director of Outpatient Recovery Centers of Metropolitan Medical Group, P.C., providers of private outpatient psychiatric services in the New York metropolitan area. Current programs are located at the Regent Hospital, New York, N.Y., and at Stony Lodge Hospital, Briarcliff Manor, New York. Dr. Washton is also Research Director of the "800-COCAINE" National Helpline based at Fair Oaks Hospital, Summit, N.J. A nationally-recognized expert in the drug abuse field, Dr. Washton established the first "cocaine helpline" in the U.S. in 1982 which later merged into the "800-COCAINE" National Helpline through collaborative efforts with Dr. Gold. Dr. Washton has published numerous articles in leading medical journals and books; has testified before special committees of the U.S. Senate, House of Representatives, and President's Commission on Organized Crime; and serves as drug abuse advisor to state, local, and federal government as well as professional sports teams and media organizations. Dr. Washton earned a bachelor's degree in psychology from New York University and received his M.A. and Ph.D. in psychology from The City University of New York.

MARK S. GOLD, M.D.

Mark S. Gold, M.D., is Director of Research at Fair Oaks Hospital, Summit, N.J./Boca Delray, Florida; The Regent Hospital, New York, N.Y.; and, Stony Lodge Hospital, Briarcliff Manor, N.Y. He is also the founder of the "800-COCAINE" National Helpline based at Fair Oaks Hospital, Summit, N.J., and author of the book "800-COCAINE" (Bantam, 1984). Dr. Gold is a nationally-recognized expert in addiction and in biological psychiatry with numerous publications in both areas. He maintains an active schedule of public speaking to high school and college students, parent groups, government bodies, and professional organizations throughout the U.S. Dr. Gold received his M.D. degree from the University of Florida College of Medicine and completed psychiatric residency training at the Yale University School of Medicine.

Table of Contents

COCAINE AND COCAINE ABUSE

1. How Cocaine Works — 1
2. Is Cocaine Addictive? — 3
3. Stages of Cocaine Abuse — 4
   Table 1: Cocaine Dependence — 5

PATIENT ASSESSMENT

4. Intake and Initial Evaluation — 6
5. Inpatient or Outpatient? — 11
6. Treatment Contracting — 12

COMPREHENSIVE OUTPATIENT TREATMENT

7. Components and Stages of Treatment — 12
8. Treatment Philosophy — 14
9. Abstinence — 15
10. Urine Testing — 16
11. Individual Counseling — 17
12. Family Involvement — 17
13. Cocaine Recovery Group — 18
14. Self-Help Groups — 20
15. Relapse Prevention Techniques — 20
16. Success Rates — 28

SPECIAL TOPICS

17. Psychiatric Issues — 28
18. Pharmacologic Treatment — 29
19. "Crack": A New Form of Cocaine Freebase — 30
20. Adolescents and Cocaine — 31
21. Women and Cocaine — 34

SUMMARY

22. Summary — 35
23. References — 37

ACKNOWLEDGEMENTS

We gratefully acknowledge the editorial assistance of Donna Boundy, M.S.W., who made preparation of this manuscript possible. We are also grateful to the clinical staff of Outpatient Recovery Centers, most notably David Zahm, Ph.D., Norma Southworth, Ph.D., and Art Greenberg, M.S.W., for their help in implementing many of the treatment techniques described in this booklet and demonstrating that these techniques really do work. Lastly, many thanks to our patients, who have taught us almost everything we know about treating addiction.

AUTHORS' NOTE

You will notice that the masculine pronoun "he" and possessive "his" are used in most sections of this pamphlet, despite the fact that a substantial number of cocaine abusers and those in treatment are female.

While we regret having to use this sentence structure, we found it preferable to clumsy repeated references to "he or she" and "him or her". The reader should remain aware that the suggestions and guidelines here apply to both male and female patients except where noted otherwise.

Cocaine Treatment Today

INTRODUCTION

The demand for treatment of cocaine abuse has increased dramatically throughout the United States in recent years. Physicians, psychologists, social workers, psychotherapists and counselors around the country report growing numbers of cocaine abusers seeking their help in overcoming one of the most ravaging addictions known to date.

Many clinicians have been caught off guard by this epidemic. Almost suddenly it seems, a largely middle class, often previously well-functioning population have begun appearing in their offices and clinics with all the earmarks of full-blown addiction. At the same time, existing literature available to the clinician contained the same misinformation that contributed to the growing abuse itself — namely, the myths that cocaine is relatively harmless and non-addicting. Because of the lack of accurate information, the special issues raised by treating this newly-dependent population, and the rapid escalation of the epidemic itself, few clinicians have acquired the expertise needed to effectively provide treatment.

The purpose of this monograph is to fill that gap: to present important new discoveries regarding the nature of cocaine dependence and to provide guidelines as well as specific strategies for the assessment, diagnosis and treatment of this patient. It focuses primarily on treatment in a structured outpatient setting — the modality that has been found to be most effective based on the authors' own clinical experience with a wide variety of cocaine-abusing patients.

While some of the approaches and techniques outlined here can be applied to the treatment of cocaine abusers in private practice, it should be noted that the best prognosis exists where a patient has the benefits of frequent contact, firm structure and limits, urine testing, and participation in a peer-support group.

HOW COCAINE WORKS

Recent findings about cocaine's activity in the brain provide important clues about the powerfully-reinforcing effects of the drug. Simply stated, the same part of the brain that reinforces basic instinctual drives (hunger, thirst, sexual desire, etc.), namely the brain's "reward center", is also activated by cocaine. Repeated introduction of cocaine into this "reward center" can cause it to replace these survival-oriented normal drives with the drive to obtain more cocaine.

Cocaine does this by causing the release of a neurotransmitter, dopamine, in the brain's nerve endings. Increased levels of dopamine (ordinarily prompted by the attainment of those survival needs) in effect "fools" the reward center into providing the "pleasure response" usually reserved for the fulfillment of those drives. It is this "pleasure response" that provides the much-touted euphoric effects of cocaine.

This explains why, for the cocaine-addicted person, obtaining and using cocaine becomes a first priority while matters related to family, career and other interests begin to take a "back seat". Cocaine has taken on the importance of a basic survival need, and the reward center of the brain has mistakenly begun to reinforce the use of cocaine.

It should be noted that the initial rise in dopamine levels in the brain caused by the introduction of cocaine is followed by a drop in dopamine below the normal level. This is what's experienced as the "crash" from cocaine, and this is what prompts the user to desire more cocaine. Repeated use of cocaine over time can cause an overall depletion in dopamine levels, resulting in the chronic depression characteristic of the cocaine addict.

Animal Experiments:

The extremely potent reinforcing effects of cocaine have been demonstrated by at least several experiments with animals:

• Animals given unlimited access to cocaine will take such massive doses that in over 95% of cases they induce in themselves fatal brain seizures and die within 30 days. The effects of cocaine appear to override the basic survival instinct.

• Hungry animals given the choice of cocaine or food invariably choose cocaine and ultimately die of starvation or toxic drug reactions.

• Animals will work to the point of total exhaustion, pressing a lever over 13,000 times to obtain a single dose of cocaine.

• Monkeys will reliably choose to press a bar that gives a high dose of cocaine followed by a painful electric shock in preference to one that gives a lower dose of cocaine with no shock.

• Sex-deprived male rhesus monkeys will choose to press a bar for cocaine injections in preference to a receptive female monkey placed in their cage.

IS COCAINE ADDICTIVE?

The debate about whether cocaine is "physically addictive" that has raged over the past decade is largely a question of semantics, or how we choose to define addiction. That controversy has focused primarily on whether cocaine produces physiological tolerance similar to other known addictive drugs and whether it produces an acute withdrawal syndrome.

The key issue here is *not* actually physiological dependence, but the fact that cocaine has access to those reward centers as described above, and can in some users set in motion an all-consuming compulsion to use the drug despite enormous adverse consequences.

This addiction, probably resulting from actual physical alterations in the user's brain chemistry, is characterized by four major features: (further detailed in Table 1)

1. Cravings and compulsions to obtain and use the drug.
2. Inability to limit or control use.
3. Continued use despite adverse consequences.
4. Denial that the problem exists.

Tolerance:

There can be little doubt that tolerance, the need to use ever increasing amounts of the drug to obtain the same effect, to cocaine does develop with repeated and chronic use. This is evidenced by the ever-increasing quantities of the drug that are needed to achieve the same desired euphoric effect, and the eventual inability to provide the "high" regardless of the amount used. Further evidence of tolerance can be found in the fact that chronic users often escalate to dosage levels that would have been toxic or fatal earlier in their use.

Withdrawal:

Although cocaine does not produce a dramatic withdrawal syndrome similar to that caused by heroin or barbiturates, the abrupt stopping of high-level doses (such as those used by heavy freebase smokers or intravenous users) can result in a variety of symptoms which last for 3 to 5 days after stopping. These include depression, irritability, restlessness, fatigue, insomnia, and intense cravings for cocaine.

While these symptoms may be viewed as a withdrawal state since they prompt renewed drug-seeking behavior, no gradual weaning from cocaine or substitute drugs are necessary. Patients should be advised to stop cocaine use abruptly and completely, as any attempt to "taper off" merely subjects the patient to the continued seduction of cocaine and makes it harder to stop.

Risk Factors:
Generally speaking, anyone is susceptible to cocaine addiction, regardless of personality structure. Since cocaine addiction may well be chemically induced, repeated use can set in motion the biologically-based craving for the drug in anyone. This is exemplified by the fact that many mature, stable, well-functioning people have become full-blown cocaine addicts even though they never intended to.

It is also true, of course, that emotionally-troubled people or people in periods of high stress, may be particularly drawn to the drug's euphoric properties and driven to repeat use. Such a person is more likely to advance from an occasional user to a regular user and thus set in motion the brain's craving response.

It is also worth noting, however, that some people may have a biological predisposition to cocaine addiction in that their brain, for as yet unknown reasons, has an exaggerated response to the drug. This is not unlike the etiology of alcoholism.

STAGES OF COCAINE ABUSE

In determining who needs treatment for cocaine abuse, it is useful to understand the chief stages of cocaine use along the progression to addiction. There are no rigid dividing lines between these stages, but the factors that motivate continued drug use in each stage differ somewhat and help to explain why some people progress from one stage to the next.

Experimental Use:
Refers to the user who has tried cocaine several times or less — chiefly out of curiosity, encouragement from others, and the drug's perceived harmlessness. If the person then somehow stops use, he will progress no further than this stage, and have no desire to resume.

Occasional/Regular Use:
This is known also as "social" or "recreational" use and refers to the user who continues to use cocaine on occasion — usually within a social setting. The factors that motivate this person to continue using the drug include the reinforcing effects of the euphoria; continued access to the drug (that is, the money to buy it or other access to a supply); perceived enhancement of performance in work, sex or other situations

that the user attributes to cocaine; and the absence of any obvious negative consequences from cocaine use up to that point.

This category contains the largest number of users, and because they have not yet suffered clear-cut negative effects, it is they who often advance the myth that cocaine is harmless. Some of these users, however, are in transition and will go on to become compulsive or dependent users.

Compulsive/Dependent/Addictive Use:
Refers to the user who no longer has control over cocaine use, but is controlled by it. The factors that motivate this person to continue using are now chiefly biochemical and behavioral, including the experience of a biologically-based craving for cocaine due to stimulation of certain brain areas, and powerful conditioning factors that make taking cocaine an habitual behavior set off by reminders and "cues" associated with the drug. See Table 1.

TABLE 1

Cocaine Dependence: Clinical Characteristics

1. *Drug Compulsion*
    - preoccupation with obtaining and using cocaine
    - persistent or periodic cravings for the drug
    - compulsive use despite eventual absence of euphoric effects
    - fears of being without cocaine
    - compulsive use of other drugs in absence of cocaine

2. *Loss of Ability to Control Use*
    - can't refuse drug when offered
    - can't self-limit the amount used
    - "binge" patterns of excessive use lasting 24 hrs. or longer
    - failed attempts to stop using

3. *Continued Use Despite Adverse Consequences*
    - medical complications: lethargy, insomnia, nasal or sinus problems, appetite disturbance, loss of sex drive, impotence
    - psychiatric complications: depression, irritability, paranoia, suicidal/homocidal ideation or gestures
    - social complications: financial, relationship, legal or job problems

4. *Denial*
    - denies that the problem exists
    - denies or downplays the seriousness of adverse effects
    - acts defensively when asked or confronted about drug use

INTAKE AND INITIAL EVALUATION

The management of initial patient contact during intake and assessment is crucial to the eventual success of treatment. The task is threefold: 1) to determine the severity of a patient's cocaine and other drug abuse and develop an appropriate treatment plan; 2) to effectively counter the patient's denial — the biggest obstacle to treatment; 3) to prepare the patient for the program's requirement of abstinence from all drugs.

Intake Information:
The severity of abuse can differ dramatically among those who seek treatment. To aid in assessment, clinicians should gather extensive information, either in person or via a questionnaire which the patient can complete prior to the initial interview. This questionnaire should elicit information in the following areas:

1. Pattern of Cocaine Use:
How often does the patient use cocaine — daily? "weekends only"? on binges? In what types of situations does he or she use — alone? with friends? with mate? at home? work? parties?

The frequency and pattern of use that becomes problematic for a user is highly individualized and impossible to predict for any one person. While generally, the more chronic and frequent the use the more severe the addiction, many "weekend only" and other sporadic users start to lose control over their drug intake, become preoccupied with thoughts about the drug and show evidence of accumulating negative effects on their health and functioning.

2. Route of Administration:
How does the patient usually use cocaine — snort? freebase? inject? How did he or she use it the first time?

Severe abuse usually develops more rapidly among freebase smokers and intravenous users because they commonly use higher doses and also use larger quantities of other drugs to counter the negative after-effects of cocaine. However, contrary to what many users believe, intranasal use ("snorting") offers no protection against addiction, as severe cocaine abuse can develop with any method of use.

3. Dosage:
On average, how many grams of cocaine does the patient use each week? At one time?

This too is highly individualized. Patients using as little as one gram per week have been clearly dependent and in need of treatment, though generally the higher the dose the more severe the addiction.

4. Impact on Psychosocial Functioning:

Does the patient miss days of work or school due to cocaine use? Reduced productivity at work? Gotten fired from a job? Gotten into debt? Gone through savings? Been arrested? Had a cocaine-related car accident? Stolen from work, family or friends? Physically hurt someone? Caused a relationship to break up? Become socially isolated? Caused arguments with spouse/mate?

Generally, the more severe the abuse, the more impaired functioning will become.

5. Impact on Sexual Functioning:

Has patient harmed his or her sexual relationship as a result of using cocaine? Had unwanted sexual encounters connected to use? Impotency? Loss of sex drive?

Cocaine is widely held to have aphrodisiac properties. Users often cite enhanced desire, cure of impotence and frigidity, increased endurance, prolonged erections and reduced inhibitions. All these initial benefits are short-lived, however. Chronic users report impotence or loss of sexual desire, and find that cocaine use may become a substitute for rather than an adjunct to sex.

6. Impact on Physical Health:

Does the patient report any of the following physical problems caused by cocaine use: Low energy? Sleep problems? Hands tremble? Runny nose? Nasal sores, bleeding? Sinus congestion? Hepatitis? Other infections? Heart "flutters"? Nausea? Chills? Seizures with loss of consciousness? Weight loss?

Where there is evidence of any serious drug-induced medical problems, the patient should receive a physical examination and appropriate laboratory tests.

7. Impact on Psychological Health:

Has the patient experienced any negative effects of cocaine on his or her mood or mental state, such as: Irritability? Short-tempered? Depression? Memory problems? Heightened suspicion of others? Anxiety/nervousness? Panic attacks? Suicidal impulses?

With chronic high-dose abuse, additional psychological effects may include extreme agitation, paranoia, personal neglect and a psychotic state indistinguishable from paranoid schizophrenia — complete with delusions and hallucinations.

8. Other Drug and Alcohol Abuse:

Has patient *ever* used or is *now* using any of the following drugs: Marijuana? Amphetamines? LSD or other psychedelics? Benzodiazepines or other tranquilizers? Barbiturates? Quaaludes? Heroin? Other opiates? Alcohol? Cigarettes/nicotine?

Many cocaine abusers are also abusing other drugs in order to counter the negative effects of the cocaine "crash". Among the most common are alcohol, marijuana and sedative-hypnotics. Heroin is also frequently used by heavy intravenous cocaine users and is the drug combination often referred to as a "speedball".

9. Treatment for Drug or Alcohol Abuse:

Has patient ever been in treatment for drug or alcohol abuse before? Where? When? Type of treatment? Ever attended Alcoholics Anonymous, Narcotics Anonymous, Pills Anonymous, or other self-help group?

10. Psychiatric History:

Has patient ever been hospitalized for psychiatric treatment? When, where and reason for treatment? Ever consulted a psychiatrist or other mental health professional?

11. Family Substance Use and Psychiatric History:

Have any family members ever been involved with illegal drugs? Any history of alcohol problems? Emotional problems? Anyone ever treated for drug addiction? Psychiatric treatment? Anyone in household use or deal drugs?

12. Strength of Drug Urges and Cravings:

An additional questionnaire or checklist may be useful for this. It should include questions such as: Do you have trouble turning down cocaine when it is offered? Do you use up your supplies of cocaine even though you try to save some? Have you been trying to stop using cocaine but find that somehow you always go back? Does the sight, thought or mention of cocaine trigger urges and cravings for the drug? Are you sometimes preoccupied with thoughts about cocaine? Do you sometimes feel an irresistible compulsion to use cocaine?

Generally, the greater the dose and chronicity of use, the stronger the drug urges and cravings in between episodes of use. The most powerful urges and cravings are often reported by free-base smokers and IV users.

Initial Interview:
During the initial interview, the above information should be reviewed with the patient. In addition, the following issues and program procedures should be addressed:

1. Reasons for Seeking Treatment:

Most cocaine abusers seek treatment only when a significant crisis has developed in their work or personal life and their own efforts to control cocaine use have failed (such as when threatened with job loss, separation or divorce, serious financial problems, severe depression, etc.). The specific reasons for seeking treatment should be given close attention in the evaluation for several reasons:

1. The patient may have consented to an initial interview only to satisfy a spouse, employer, etc. and have little intention of actually entering treatment.
2. He or she may see the problem as belonging to the spouse, employer or other person who pressured him to apply and not see the cocaine use as a problem at all.
3. Addressing specific reasons for seeking treatment can help pierce the denial most patients come in with.

2. Expectations of Treatment:

Many patients apply for treatment with the expectation that they will be able to return to "controlled" or "social" cocaine use. In order to help the patient counter this denial of his problem during the early stages of treatment, it is often useful to refer back to information collected during the initial interview.

3. Life Events:

It is also important to review in detail the patient's history of escalating cocaine use to uncover possible connections with other problems or life events. This account may reveal a history of "self-medication" for boredom, stress relief, depression, sexual problems, career crisis, difficulty in relationships or other personal problems.

4. Support Systems:

Assessment of the cocaine abuser should also address the patient's general lifestyle and available support network as these may affect recovery and/or contribute to relapse. Information should be gathered about the following:

1. Does patient have the support of significant others, such as spouse, other family members or friends?

2. Does patient have a social network of friends who do not use drugs?

3. Does patient come into frequent contact with others who use (through job, dealing drugs, etc.)?

4. Does patient have alternative sources of gratification with which to fill the gaps created by stopping cocaine use, such as interests in sports, hobbies, etc.?

5. *Feelings About Entering Treatment:*

Many cocaine abusers seeking help have never been in that position before and, in fact, are often accustomed to being "the one in control". It is very difficult for a patient who considers himself "successful" and who may indeed have managed his life fairly well up to now to admit being "powerless" over cocaine use. There is also a great deal of fear about confidentiality and about the stigma attached to seeking help in a drug abuse treatment program. It is important to discuss these issues during the initial assessment.

6. *Beginning Abstinence:*

During the initial contact with the patient, the program's requirement of abstinence from all drug and alcohol use must be discussed. Patients are often relieved to learn that there will be limits placed on them in this way. Patients must be exhorted to discard all remaining drug supplies and paraphernalia upon returning home and to sever relationships with drug dealers immediately. If money is owed to a dealer, it should be paid off as soon as possible, even if this requires taking a loan, and the payment should be delivered by someone other than the patient, such as a messenger.

7. *Obtain Urine Sample:*

Testing the urine obtained from an initial visit should serve to confirm the history provided by the patient. It can also reveal other drug use which the patient is denying and therefore help to set the stage for honesty and total abstinence.

8. *Physical Examination:*

A physical examination and clinical lab tests should be included in the assessment procedure if there are questions about the patient's health status — especially for heavy freebase smokers and i.v. users. While serious medical complications are fairly uncommon in most cocaine abusers, freebase smokers may exhibit upper respiratory problems (chest congestion, coughing, wheezing), and i.v. users may have systemic infections (hepatitis, endocarditis), or abscesses at injection sites. Some intranasal users report chronic rhinorrhea, sinus congestion, nasal sores or bleeding and headaches.

INPATIENT OR OUTPATIENT?

Based on the initial assessment of a patient, the first critical decision in treatment is whether or not the patient needs to be hospitalized. Fortunately, hospitalization is not routinely required, for in most cases cocaine can be stopped abruptly without medical risk or a dramatic withdrawal syndrome, and no substitute drugs or gradual weaning from cocaine are needed or even advised. There are, however, some circumstances in which hospitalization is clearly indicated.

Criteria for Hospitalization:

Initial hospitalization is indicated for those with the following characteristics:

1. Heavy users whose drug compulsion is uncontrollable, usually heavy freebase and i.v. users.
2. Those who require a medically-supervised detoxification from physical addiction to another drug, such as alcohol or barbiturates.
3. Those with severe medical or psychiatric complications.
4. Those with severe psychosocial impairment (unable to care for themselves, etc.).
5. Those who lack family and social supports.
6. Those who have failed in outpatient treatment.

Role of Hospitalization:

The major objectives of inpatient treatment should be to break the cycle of compulsive drug use, address related and coexisting problems, and strengthen the patient's motivation and skills for remaining abstinent after hospital discharge. Hospitalization should be seen as only the first step in a more comprehensive recovery plan that must include outpatient aftercare treatment. Permanent abstinence following inpatient treatment alone is highly unlikely.

Advantages of Outpatient Treatment:

Outpatient treatment has many advantages for the cocaine abuser who does not need hospitalization. In addition to substantially lower costs, a major clinical advantage is greater patient acceptability. Patients often have much less resistance to entering an outpatient program, and many state that they would not be entering treatment at all if hospitalization were the only option. The reasons are fairly obvious: Outpatient treatment is less disruptive to the patient's job and family life and less stigmatizing than being hospitalized for a drug problem.

The advantages of outpatient treatment may extend beyond the patient himself. Because cocaine abusers might accept outpatient treatment at an earlier stage of their addiction than they would hospitalization, incalculable damage to them, their families and other victims of their drug problem may be avoided.

TREATMENT CONTRACTING

At the end of the initial interview, a written treatment contract should be drawn up to clarify and concretize treatment requirements. The contract should specify the following:

1. That the patient immediately discontinue use of all mood-altering substances.
2. That the patient remain in treatment for no less than 6-12 months since this is the minimum amount of time needed to begin a solid recovery and promote long-lasting changes in lifestyle and behavior.
3. That a urine sample be provided whenever requested.
4. That a severe relapse may necessitate immediate hospitalization.
5. That designated family members and/or significant others can be involved in the treatment, contacted in the event of a relapse or premature termination from treatment, and to discuss treatment programs.

While these are the "bottom line" requirements for outpatient treatment contracts, it is important that the overall plan reflect the patient's own particular history and treatment needs. No single treatment approach is optimal in all cases.

The contract must be reviewed by, and be agreeable to, the patient in order to be effective. It is advisable to also review the contract with the spouse or other person significant to the patient's treatment so that they can both understand and support it.

COMPONENTS AND STAGES OF TREATMENT

A comprehensive outpatient treatment program, whether serving as primary treatment or as an aftercare pro-

gram following hospitalization, should include the following components:
1. A requirement of complete abstinence from cocaine and all drug and alcohol use.
2. Frequent patient contact with program.
3. Frequent urine testing.
4. Group counseling.
5. Education on preventing relapse.
6. Family involvement.

Treatment is best provided by a team including professionals with expertise in managing addictive disorders and recovering counselors with at least two years of abstinence.

Stages of Treatment:
In our outpatient program, treatment is roughly divided into four phases, each of which focuses on specific tasks in the recovery process. There are no rigid dividing lines between the successive phases and patients progress through these stages at differing rates. The program is outlined below:

PHASE I: STOPPING ALL DRUG USE
1. Initial 30-day period
2. Individual counseling (1/2 hour) several times weekly
3. Drug education meetings with family 1 × wk.
4. Goals:
   a. Stop all drug use
   b. Break through denial
   c. Learn to anticipate and handle drug urges
   d. Form initial support network

PHASE II: PREVENTING RELAPSE
1. Next 6-12 months
2. Individual and/or family counseling 1 × wk.
3. Cocaine Recovery Group 2 × wk.
4. Goals:
   a. Learn to recognize early warning signs of relapse
   b. Counter "selective forgetting" and stop idealizing the cocaine "high"
   c. Prevent slips from becoming full-blown relapses
   d. Learn to cope with stress and have fun without drugs
   e. Avoid high-risk situations
   f. Begin to form positive social relationships

PHASE III: PREPARING FOR LONG-TERM ABSTINENCE
1. Next 6-12 months
2. Individual counseling if indicated
3. "Advanced" Cocaine Recovery Group 1 × wk.
4. Goals:
   a. Enhance personal relationships and self-esteem
   b. Counteract "flare-up" periods of denial and overconfidence
   c. Address issues of "arrested maturity"
   d. Strengthen commitment to drug-free living
   e. Begin to realize plans, goals and aspirations

PHASE IV: FOLLOW-UP
1. Periodic visits
2. More frequent visits during high stress or "flare-up" periods
3. Continued participation in self-help group (such as Cocaine Anonymous)

TREATMENT PHILOSOPHY

A critical element in effective outpatient treatment is the existence of a consistent treatment philosophy upon which the program's various components are built. That which the authors have found most effective includes the following points:

1. The goals of treatment are twofold: To enable the patient to become and remain drug-free, and to help him or her develop a reasonably satisfying lifestyle without drugs.

2. Cocaine addiction is a form of chemical dependency and addictive disease.

3. Cocaine addiction must be treated as a primary disorder and not merely as a symptom of underlying psychopathology — even where the latter coexists.

4. The cocaine-addicted patient is not responsible for the existence of the addictive disease but *is* responsible for his or her recovery and behavior.

5. Many of the other behavioral, psychological and social difficulties presented by the patient are the result of cocaine use rather than the cause of it.

6. Abstinence from cocaine and all drugs is a prerequisite for effective treatment — not an end result.

7. A return to "controlled use" of cocaine is unrealistic and dangerous.

8. Recovery is possible and life enhancing.

ABSTINENCE

From Cocaine:
The treatment must require immediate and complete stopping of cocaine use. A treatment goal of returning to "occasional" use is not only unrealistic but potentially dangerous for anyone who has been dependent on cocaine. Likewise, a goal of reducing rather than discontinuing cocaine altogether is unacceptable for even rare use will eventually lead back to heavy use and additional negative consequences for the patient.

The benefits of psychotherapy and drug education can only be realized during a period of prolonged abstinence. Some of the lack of success reported by private therapists working with cocaine addicts stems from a reluctance to be directive on this issue. Relying exclusively on psychotherapy and the acquisition of insight to bring an eventual end to the drug use fails to recognize that the drug addiction is a primary disorder and ignores the powerful compulsive nature of addictive behavior. Unfortunately, this posture leads the therapist to serve as an enabler of the patient's continued drug use.

From All Other Drugs, Including Alcohol:
Abstinence from all mood-altering drugs, including alcohol and marijuana, is important in order to maximize the benefits of treatment and minimize the possibility of relapse. The major goals of treatment must be to develop a reasonably satisfying drug free lifestyle and to develop ways of coping without resorting to mood-altering chemicals of any kind.

The majority of cocaine abusers (68% in a sample of Hotline callers) report using other drugs, particularly to alleviate the unpleasant after-effects of cocaine. Most common are alcohol, sleeping pills, tranquilizers and opiates. Convincing new patients to give up these other drugs is one of the hardest jobs facing the clinician.

Many cocaine abusers particularly resist abstaining from alcohol, stating they have had no problem with this substance in the past and would like to continue "social" drinking. The clinician must emphasize that complete abstinence offers the best insurance against relapse based on the experience of many before them in treatment, stressing the following points:

1. Other drug use is often subliminally associated with cocaine, having been used together repeatedly in the past. Use of the associated drug will trigger urges and cravings for cocaine — making abstinence harder.

2. The "disinhibiting" effect of any drug also makes relapse more likely, undermining the patient's own desire to recover.

3. While trying to be abstinent from cocaine, patients often switch to other drugs, merely substituting one for another. The goal, again, is to have a satisfying life without drugs.

4. Patients often have a more serious problem with other drug use than recognized.

URINE TESTING

Throughout the entire course of treatment, the patient's urine should be tested at least 2-3 times per week for cocaine and all other commonly abused drugs (e.g. opiates, barbiturates, benzodiazepines, amphetamines, marijuana, PCP, etc.). The urine sample should be obtained under staff supervision — patients must not be allowed to bring in a sample on their own, as the nature of addictive behavior leads many patients to substitute samples, etc.

Despite mutual trust and a strong therapeutic alliance between patient and clinician, urine testing is always necessary because of the re-emerging denial and self-deceit characteristic of the chemical dependency problem. Clinicians who leave out this essential treatment component are likely to become enablers of the patient's continuing drug use.

It must be emphasized that the purpose of urine testing is *NOT* to catch the patient in a lie. Rather, urine testing is a valuable treatment tool that helps the patient break through denial, gain self-control over drug-use urges, and document his progress in treatment. It is the authors' experience that patients do not object to urine screenings and often state that they feel more secure knowing the clinician can't be fooled.

It must be stipulated at the outset of treatment, in the patient's contract, that there will be consequences for drug-positive urines. It is impossible to specify here, however, the exact number of positive urines or "slips" that should result in a patient's hospitalization, or precisely which patients should be suspended from the program altogether. These decisions are highly individualized clinical decisions for which there is no pat formula. Furthermore, it would be a gross mistake to inform a patient in advance the exact number of positive urines that will result in such consequences. Given the nature of addictive disease, most patients would rationalize that it is then "o.k." to use cocaine again that number of times.

In general, however, although a rare "slip" might be anticipated (though not "permitted" as such), any emerging pattern of regular or frequent drug use should lead to revision of the treatment plan (more frequent visits, more urine tests, and hospitalization if other efforts fail).

Patients should be encouraged to report any instances of drug use before it is detected in the urine so that discussion of the circumstances can take place — maximizing the possible gains from the mistake and preventing a "slip" from becoming a full-blown relapse.

The standard type of urine test used by most laboratories, "thin layer chromatography" (TLC), is not sensitive enough to be useful in an outpatient cocaine abuse treatment program. This method of screening is capable of detecting the use of cocaine only up to 24 hours after each use, and may show a high rate of "false negative" results (i.e., the test shows that no cocaine is present when it actually is).

Enzyme-immunoassay (EIA) or radio-immunoassay (RIA) techniques, while slightly more expensive, are far superior for this use, detecting cocaine with greater accuracy and reliability for up to 72 hours after last use.

INDIVIDUAL COUNSELING

Throughout the first phases of treatment, brief (1/2 hour) individual counseling sessions should be scheduled frequently. These should be reality-oriented, focusing on practical techniques for achieving and maintaining abstinence and should provide direction, feedback and encouragement. Psychoanalytic psychotherapy is contraindicated at this stage of recovery because the feelings that surface during this kind of exploration may be too threatening for a patient struggling to remain drug-free.

Once a patient has demonstrated consistent abstinence for a period of months, a more insight-oriented therapy may be begun if a patient so wishes and is receptive to this method, but only in addition to participation in a Cocaine Recovery Group. Individual sessions now could focus more on issues pertaining to relationships, sexual functioning, self-esteem, etc.

FAMILY INVOLVEMENT

It is very important to involve close family members and especially the spouse/partner (or parent if patient is adolescent) in the treatment. Well-intentioned family members often unwittingly function as enablers by making excuses for the cocaine abuser, providing money for the drug, or trying to spare the patient from suffering the consequences of his or her behavior. They need instruction and guidance in how to deal with the cocaine abuser in a way that will support and not sabotage recovery. They also need an opportunity to deal with their own feelings of anger, blame, guilt and victimization so as to minimize any family stress which could itself contribute to relapse and treatment failure.

During the assessment period, it is advisable to meet with the patient and family (or significant others) to formulate the treatment contract. When family members can be helped to understand the basic goals and strategies of treatment and can participate in the process from the start, they often lend more consistent support to it. They also can provide additional information about the patient's drug use and other behavior.

During Phases I and II of the patient's treatment, families often benefit from attending a Family Education and Support Group held at least once weekly as part of the program. Here they join other families to learn about cocaine, addictive behavior, concepts of "enabling", etc. They also obtain the needed peer support and identification from others present and can begin to resolve some of their own anger or guilt connected with the patient's drug problem.

Cocaine-abusing spouses should be required to also enter treatment, as part of a treatment contract that provides the best insurance against relapse for the patient requesting treatment. If the spouse in this case insists on being able to discontinue cocaine use without treatment, he or she should be required to come in for regular urine screenings. The clinician should maintain a firm stand on this issue. To ignore the likelihood of relapse if the recovering person continues to live with someone using cocaine is to collude with the patient's own denial.

COCAINE RECOVERY GROUP

After approximately 30 days of complete abstinence from all drug use, the patient should be inducted into an ongoing Cocaine Recovery Group that meets at least twice weekly — an invaluable component of outpatient treatment. It is best if this group is co-facilitated by a professional therapist with expertise in treating addictive disorders and a recovering counselor with several years of abstinence and supervised clinical experience.

Each group should include patients in different stages of recovery ranging from newcomers to those with six or more months of abstinence. This mixture allows new patients the benefit of immediate exposure to positive role models and proof that recovery is indeed possible. It also provides more senior members with a healthy reminder of their own experiences in the early stage of recovery.

This group serves several important functions. First, it promotes rapid identification with others having a similar addiction problem, reducing the intense feelings of "uniqueness", isolation and shame often suffered by newcomers. Second, the positive peer support in the group helps reinforce patients' motivation to stay drug-free — reducing ambivalence and countering denial and resistance. Third, the group serves as a forum for education about the nature of addictive disease and teaches specific techniques to prevent relapse.

Group discussion frequently focuses on accepting that one has a chemical dependency problem; on feelings, addictive thinking and drug-urges that surface during recovery; on drug-free alternatives for dealing with stress and having fun; and other ways that members are changing behavior, lifestyle, and attitudes in order to achieve long-lasting recovery (relapse prevention techniques).

Ground Rules:

It is important that a Cocaine Recovery Group maintain certain ground rules, including the following:

1. The content of group discussions and identity of members must be held in strict confidence.

2. No one is permitted to attend a group session while under the influence of drugs or alcohol.

3. Reliable and punctual attendance at meetings is required to maintain membership.

4. Any member who offers drugs to another is permanently and immediately expelled from the group.

5. Romantic and/or sexual involvement among group members is strongly discouraged.

In addition, members agree to provide a supervised urine sample before every group session.

Resistance to Group:

Many new patients are strongly resistant to the idea of joining a recovery group because they have concerns about confidentiality and are reluctant to share personal problems with strangers. Our experience indicates that despite these negative expectations, however, most patients adjust rapidly to the group within the first few sessions and respond very positively to their newly-found peer-support network. Still, there are a small number of patients who are not clinically appropriate for a recovery group, including those with serious psychiatric disturbance and those who object so strongly to entering the group that insisting on it would likely have a destructive influence on both the individual patient and the group.

"Senior" Recovery Group:
By the time patients have achieved 9-12 months of abstinence, we have found that the initial recovery group begins to have diminishing usefulness for them. At that point, introduction to a "senior" recovery group helps to keep the recovery process moving forward.

The senior group provides a forum in which longer-term recovery issues can be dealt with more effectively. The focus of sessions will often shift from early abstinence issues to topics such as relationships, self-esteem, job/career problems, and other personal matters which can be discussed more freely when drug urges and the immediate threat of unpredictable relapse have diminished.

SELF-HELP GROUPS

Rather than competing with or running counter to the treatment approach of a structured outpatient program, "outside" self-help groups such as Cocaine Anonymous actually compliment it — enhancing therapeutic success and providing an invaluable and unique source of information and emotional support for program patients. In fact, for many patients, participation in such a self-help group is essential to their long-term recovery and remains a continuing source of support long after treatment has ended.

Many cocaine abusers in treatment feel "unique" and isolated in their struggle to remain abstinent. The powerful drug urges and cravings they experience seem to them to be something "no one else can understand". Attendance at Cocaine Anonymous meetings, however, helps to reduce this sense of isolation as patients can usually readily identify with what is shared there by other recovering cocaine abusers.

Cocaine Anonymous is modeled after Alcoholics Anonymous (A.A.) and Narcotics Anonymous (N.A.), utilizing the same 12 steps of recovery which include admitting one's powerlessness over drugs (in this case specifically cocaine) and the need for total abstinence to arrest the disease of chemical dependency. The C.A. peer-support network is available around the clock at no cost to anyone who wants to stop using cocaine, and chapters are proliferating rapidly in many areas of the country. In places where C.A. chapters do not exist, patients should be encouraged to attend A.A. or N.A. meetings.

RELAPSE PREVENTION TECHNIQUES

In the past, the drug abuse field has focused too much on getting the addict off the drug and too little on keeping him off. Our approach to outpatient treatment includes the use of specific relapse prevention techniques, some of which have been adapted from the earlier work of Marlatt with alcoholics.

Patients need to be educated about certain attitudes, thinking patterns and behavior that are characteristic of addiction so that they can anticipate the pitfalls most patients face during recovery. By bringing these pitfalls or "mind-traps" to their attention, patients learn to avoid or deal with them and replace them with constructive recovery-enhancing behaviors. We list here the various pitfalls and also specific skills that can be taught patients to aid them in recovery.

Pitfalls in Recovery:

1. Self-Sabotage ("Set-ups")

Patients who are headed for relapse typically engage in a series of self-sabotaging acts, "setting themselves up" for a return to drug use. Often the "set-up" includes putting themselves in a high-risk situation, one where they will be tempted to use drugs, while denying (even to themselves) that it does involve that risk.

Examples of "set-ups" include re-initiating contact with drug-using friends, deciding to "pass by" some of the places associated with buying or using drugs, or "accidentally" placing oneself in a high-risk situation such as a party where cocaine is being used. Another kind of "set-up" is allowing stressful circumstances to build up until one feels "justified" in using cocaine to cope with them or as a "well-deserved reward".

There are some warning signs that often appear when a patient is beginning to engage in self-sabotage. These include increased fighting and disharmony with spouse and others at home or work; a build-up of financial or work pressures, and other personal problems. Often this is the first time the patient is faced with "everyday" problems while not using cocaine since the start of recovery. Unconsciously the patient may be yearning for this "way out" or "relief" again and hence the self-sabotage begins.

Denial figures largely in self-sabotage. The clinician, therefore, must be able to spot the warning signs and appropriately alert and confront the patient when this may be occurring. The Cocaine Recovery Group is useful in this process too. About 3-4 months into recovery is a particularly vulnerable time, as this is when many patients become overconfident and begin to believe they can go to parties where cocaine is used and resist, resume relationships with friends who use, etc.

Patients can also be taught the early warning signs that often precede self-sabotage and relapse so they can begin to catch themselves. A heightened awareness of how their use of rationalization and denial is setting them up for relapse is of enormous help to patients throughout the course of treatment and this kind of insight should be encouraged.

2. Idealizing the Cocaine "High"
("Selective Forgetting")

After 1-2 months of abstinence, many patients begin idealizing the cocaine "high" again — remembering only the pleasurable and euphoric effects of the drug. The negative consequences of its effects on their health, marriages and jobs, etc. begin to fade into the past and lose the strong motivating force they once had. This continued "romanticizing" of cocaine experiences and selective "forgetting" of the numerous adverse effects tends to heighten the allure of the drug and primes the patient for eventual relapse.

Although their search for euphoria has ended in the opposite (dysphoria, depression, etc.), the users thoughts and associations to cocaine still center primarily on the drug's pleasurable effects — the exhilarating high, the sexual stimulation, the feeling of confidence and energy. Denial reemerges as patients selectively forget the car accidents, the family breakup, the many job losses, the need to borrow money to pay daily expenses despite high salaries, etc. It is this selective memory (also called "euphoric recall") that heightens the patient's ambivalence about giving up cocaine entirely.

This selective forgetting usually occurs when the patient is under stress and the desire to immediately "medicate" bad feelings or seek relief is strong, since cocaine abusers are conditioned to think first of cocaine for relief. In fact, the tendency to idealize cocaine is usually strongest exactly when a patient is on the verge of relapse. It is as if the selective forgetting process is in the service of the patient's denial, helping him to set himself up for relapse.

To counteract selective forgetting, the patient must be reminded repeatedly, throughout the course of treatment, of the numerous drug-related consequences that finally compelled him to seek help. The notion that the euphoria can be recaptured without the "down side" of drug-induced consequences must be countered with reality whenever patients nostalgically reminisce about the cocaine "high". Help patients formulate a more realistic appraisal of the way cocaine use has affected their lives.

Recommend that patients keep ugly reminders of their experiences with cocaine as visible as possible. For example, one patient did not fix a smashed car fender for six months so that every time he used his expensive car, he'd see that ugly crumpled fender and be reminded of what had happened to him while on cocaine.

Continued participation in a Cocaine Recovery Group also helps to counter selective forgetting as the experiences shared by newcomers often remind senior group members again of the ravages of cocaine dependence.

3. Testing Control:

After a period of initial abstinence, many patients begin to harbor the fantasy that they can now return to using cocaine in a limited way without losing control. Or, they may accept the need to remain completely abstinent from cocaine but want to test control over alcohol or marijuana. As mentioned earlier, use of these other drugs impedes the recovery process too and may well lead to a cocaine relapse.

Having the belief that they have acquired enough "strength" to use cocaine or other drugs in a limited way without losing control is always a clear indication of the patient's continuing denial and is one of the most common predictions of relapse. Yet this desire or plan is usually hidden and not verbalized by the patient without active prompting from the clinician.

This "mind trap" can be best countered by informing the patient ahead of time that this desire to test control occurs in most patients and is itself a symptom of addictive disease, and by reiterating and explaining that a return to controlled use is not possible once a person has crossed the line into addictive or compulsive drug use.

4. From "Slip" Into Relapse:
(The "Abstinence Violation Effect")

The Abstinence Violation Effect, as described by Marlatt and Gordon, is one of the most useful concepts in relapse prevention. It refers to the defeatist reaction patients often have when they "slip" and violate a period of abstinence. The defeatist reaction goes something like "Now that I've blown it (recovery), I might as well go all the way". This way of thinking turns what could have been an isolated incident into a full-blown relapse.

When the abstinence violation effect is occurring, a "slip" sets off a complex of negative feelings, including:

1. Profound feelings of failure and an expectation of continued failure from this point on.

2. A feeling that all progress up to that point has been lost.

3. Feelings of guilt, remorse and self-loathing for having "given in to temptation", and an attribution of the "slip" to personal weakness and lack of willpower.

4. Feelings of identity confusion because the renewed drug use is inconsistent with one's most recent self-image as an abstainer. ("I must have been a big fraud in treatment — this is the real 'me'.")

If these negative reactions are not prevented or short-circuited effectively, the likelihood that any single slip will escalate into a full-blown destructive relapse and lead the patient to drop out of treatment, becomes much greater.

As with all the other pitfalls of recovery, patients benefit enormously from being informed ahead of time about this common reaction to slips and from being prepared with a specific action plan to counteract it. The patient and his family should be told that "slips" do sometimes occur during recovery and do not automatically mean that treatment has failed. It is an unrealistic expectation that a recovering person can be guaranteed a lifetime of total abstinence simply by entering treatment. Again, it is important for the patient and his family to gain an understanding of the powerful grip of addictive disease with its predictable symptoms of denial and rationalization.

While it is essential to recognize the possibility of "slips" in order to minimize their destructive consequences, this should not be construed by the patient as permission to use drugs occasionally. Total abstinence is still the major treatment goal (and in fact the only way recovery can truly occur), but slips and relapses must not be allowed to nullify or derail the recovery process.

The patient should be taught to reconceptualize a "slip" as a single, independent event — a temporary "rough spot" on the road to recovery — not a total nullification of progress. The occurrence of any "slip" is likely to elicit feelings of personal failure and weakness, accompanied by thoughts like "I'm just a helpless addict so why continue to fight it." This is part of the "mind trap" that can lure the patient back into full relapse with all the negative consequences of cocaine use again. These thoughts and feelings, while they appear as "fact" at the time to the patient, are merely rationalizations in the service of his addictive disease, or "the disease talking".

Lastly, the patient should be assisted in devising alternative coping strategies for handling any slip, including the plan to "put on the brakes" and immediately contact someone in his support network. The patient should also be encouraged to tell his counselor or therapist as soon as possible when a slip has occurred, so that the most can be learned from it through discussion.

The clinician should ask nonjudgmental questions in going over the slip, such as "How could you have avoided it?", "If this same sequence of events occurs next week, can you think of how you could handle it differently so it would not lead again to drug use?", etc.

New Skills for Recovery:

1. Avoiding High-Risk Situations:

Inevitably, patients will encounter high-risk situations — situations likely to increase their temptation to use cocaine and other drugs — during the course of recovery. An important component of relapse prevention, then, is to teach patients how to anticipate, avoid and cope with such situations.

High-risk situations include any that involve "people, places or things" formerly associated with the use of cocaine or other drugs. Going to a party where there is a possibility cocaine will be available or used, for example, is undoubtedly a high-risk situation.

It is very difficult for some patients to accept the fact that they can no longer socialize with cocaine users if they want to remain abstinent. Participation in a Cocaine Recovery Group, however, is useful in helping a patient break through his denial about the risk certain situations contain and get support for avoiding such "people, places and things".

One particularly high-risk situation is, of course, having any contact with a dealer. Patients must be instructed to break off relationships with dealers and to pay off any money owed them immediately upon entering treatment — even if a loan must be taken out to do so. Otherwise, it is likely that the high-risk contact will continue between patient and dealer.

Patients should also be advised not to handle cocaine or help anyone obtain it, and to avoid specific places and persons associated with cocaine use and anyone who offers cocaine or uses it in their presence. Patients should be helped to anticipate high-risk situations by "imagining" several high-risk situations likely to arise in their daily lives and devise strategies for coping with or avoiding them.

2. Dealing With Urges and Cravings:

The conditioned cravings set off by cocaine are extremely strong and hard to extinguish. Patients must be helped to anticipate and cope with these sometimes sudden and powerful drug cravings that inevitably occur during recovery.

Often the cravings are triggered predictably by specific environmental stimuli (i.e., people, places and things) previously associated with cocaine, by certain internal feeling states such as boredom, depression and fatigue that have been followed by drug use in the past, or even by happy events (promotion, wedding, etc.) which would have previously been accompanied by celebrating with cocaine. Cravings can also occur seemingly "out of nowhere" without prior warning — touched off by, for example, the mere mention of cocaine on television or in a magazine article.

Patients often erroneously conclude that having a strong, unexpected drug urge means that treatment is not working for them. This, in turn, may prompt the patient to impulsively terminate treatment. It is essential, therefore, to warn patients about drug cravings and to emphasize that they should be expected to occur as a normal and predictable part of the recovery process.

Another common misconception about drug urges that should be addressed is the belief that once a craving begins it will only keep building and that it will only be satisfied with drug use. Patients should learn that cravings and urges are always temporary and tend to reach a peak of intensity within 1-2 hours in most instances. Using cocaine during a drug urge serves only to increase the strength of future urges, whereas "riding it out" each time will decrease the power of the urges in the future.

Drug urges can be short-circuited by one or more substitute activities, and patients should learn these and plan what they will do when hit with an urge or craving. Patients should learn to react by:

1. Removing oneself from access to drugs or people that would give them drugs.

2. Leave the place or situation in which the drug urge is occurring.

3. Immediately phone or meet with a member of their support network — assigned counselor/therapist or an abstinent member of their family or their recovery group.

Another technique that can be useful is that of mentally detaching oneself from the drug urge so as to examine the feeling from the vantage point of a dispassionate outside observer. Relaxation and other stress-reduction techniques may also be helpful. The goal in all of these interventions is to block or eliminate the impulse to satisfy the drug urge.

It is always best if patients devise these alternative action plans in advance of experiencing a drug urge rather than trying to do this while in the grips of it. Planning ahead and rehearsing alternative behaviors is crucial.

To help patients better understand and cope with drug urges, they should also be taught the role of conditioning factors in addictive behavior. Discussions should include:

1. The mechanics of environmental "triggers" — how they occur.

2. How deconditioning can work by reducing the strength of drug urges that are not followed by drug use.

3. How drug-seeking behavior can be thwarted in its earliest stage before it builds up too much strength to be stopped.

Explaining these conditioning phenomena can help greatly to relieve unnecessary guilt and counterproductive feelings of uniqueness and shame. However, the importance of taking responsibility for *how* one deals with the drug urges must be emphasized.

3. Building a Satisfying Lifestyle

One of the most common rationalizations for relapse is the belief that one's desire to indulge is "justified". This rationalization usually results from feeling stressed, overworked, deprived, or otherwise in need of relief from the demands of everyday life. Many cocaine abusers have been "workaholics" whose daily lifestyles are severely out of balance. Often cocaine use has been the only form of self-gratification they have allowed themselves on any regular basis. Achieving a more balanced lifestyle, then, is essential to reduce the potential for relapse.

Issues to be addressed with the patient around "lifestyle" include the following:

1. Establishing a regular schedule of exercise and recreation.

2. Learning to have fun without drugs.

3. Learning to reduce stress without drugs.

4. Forming a reliable peer-support network of non-drug-using friends.

5. Improving nutrition.

6. Improving interpersonal relationships.

7. Examining and realigning values, priorities and goals.

Addressing these issues regarding lifestyle help not only to reduce stress for the patient but also to instill a feeling of greater control over one's life. These issues can best be addressed both in the Recovery Group and through individual counseling.

SUCCESS RATES

Success rates in an outpatient program will depend, of course, upon a variety of factors including the severity of patient's abuse, the patient's motivation to become drug-free, and the extent to which the program meets the patient's most critical needs — namely for structure, accountability, education and peer-support. The highest success rates can be expected in those patients who have a history of good functioning before cocaine use, a genuine acceptance that their chemical dependency problem does exist, and an acceptance of the need for total abstinence and lifestyle change.

In our highly structured and intensive outpatient program, we have found that over 65% of patients complete the 6-12-month program and over 75% of that group are still drug-free at 1-2-year follow-up.

PSYCHIATRIC ISSUES

Evaluation for the presence of psychiatric illness is an essential component of the assessment process. While the incidence of severe psychiatric disorders among cocaine abusers appears to be relatively low and many are fairly high-functioning individuals with no previous history of addiction or significant psychopathology, some do exhibit clearly definable psychiatric disorders by history and persisting symptoms, including depressive or bipolar disorders, anxiety disorders or severe narcissistic or borderline personality disorders.

It is essential to allow a sufficient post-cocaine recovery period (at least 2-3 weeks) before making a definitive psychiatric diagnosis or introducing psychotropic medication. The reason for this is the pharmacologic effects of cocaine may generate behavioral patterns and affective states that closely resemble symptoms of such psychiatric illnesses as depression, bipolar disorders, attention deficit disorders and anxiety disorders. Similarly, the acute after-effects of cocaine ("crash") and the chronic effects of habitual use tend to resemble symptoms of depression, including anergia, sleep and appetite disturbance, sexual disinterest, and negative mood states. These depressive symptoms are not usually responsive to antidepressant medication and often dissipate without medical intervention within a week or two of stopping cocaine use.

Cocaine-Induced Psychosis:

Some chronic high-dose cocaine abusers (especially heavy free-base smokers and i.v. users) exhibit a transient cocaine-induced psychosis which is virtually indistinguishable from paranoid schizophrenia. Symptoms include delusions, hallucinations, deterioration in personal care, marked confusion, and sometimes violent or suicidal behavior. This cocaine-induced psychosis tends to be self-limiting in most cases, with psychotic symptoms disappearing within 2-5 days after ending drug use.

In a small number of cases, however, chronic high-level cocaine use appears to precipitate an underlying psychosis that persists despite stopping the drug abuse. If psychosis persists beyond several days or if the patient becomes increasingly difficult to manage, hospitalization and introduction of neuroleptics may be needed. After a stabilization period, further evaluation can be carried out to determine whether the psychosis persists.

Dual Diagnosis:

In cases where there is a genuine dual diagnosis of psychiatric illness and chemical dependency, both problems must be treated. It is nonetheless imperative that the drug abuse problem continue to be dealt with as a *primary disorder* and not merely as a symptom of the psychiatric illness.

In order to avoid unrealistic or distorted expectations, patients who receive psychotropic medication should be informed that the medication is to treat their psychiatric disorder and not to prevent relapse to drug use. The medication cannot be seen as a substitute for the lifestyle change and other treatment efforts that are essential to recovery.

PHARMACOLOGIC TREATMENT

There is no definitive evidence that antidepressants, lithium, amino acids or other psychotropic agents block the cocaine euphoria, ameliorate post-cocaine symptoms, or eliminate craving for cocaine. There is no known cocaine antagonist and no medication that has been shown to prevent relapse, despite earlier claims which have not been replicated. If such medications were found they might indeed be helpful, especially in extreme or intractable cases where psychological interventions alone have failed.

Recent trials with bromocriptine, a dopamine agonist, suggest the potential use of this drug in eliminating urges and cravings for cocaine during the immediate post-drug abstinence period. Bromocriptine may decrease early treatment dropouts which may be due to a covert withdrawal syndrome. However, the clinical efficacy of bromocriptine in treating cocaine abusers remains to be determined, through carefully controlled studies.

"CRACK": A NEW FORM OF COCAINE FREEBASE

Increasing numbers of patients report using a new form of cocaine, the street name of which is "crack" or "rock". This is a ready-to-smoke form of cocaine freebase, or freebase "rocks", being sold at relatively low prices. Because its "packaging" and pricing makes this potent form of cocaine available and attractive to larger numbers of users — including teenagers — its appearance marks a very dangerous new development in the cocaine epidemic.

These freebase "rocks" look like beige or slightly brownish clumps of sugar and are typically sold in small plastic vials at a price of about $10 for a 100 mg rock. Like other freebase, these "rocks" are typically smoked in a glass pipe using a butane torch, or put into a tobacco or marijuana cigarette. This new form of cocaine makes it possible for a user to smoke freebase without going through a dangerous and involved process of extracting the potent freebase from its parent compound, cocaine hydrochloride powder. For the users of "crack", as with other freebase smoking, it means a more rapid, more powerful, and more destructive addiction as compared to snorting the white cocaine powder.

The popularity of crack seems to be increasing with amazing speed. No statistics are available yet on the prevalence of crack use in the U.S., although the problem has already surfaced in over 16 major cities and their adjoining suburbs. Among callers to our "800-COCAINE" National Hotline, nearly one-third of all cocaine users report addiction to crack. Although most of these crack users are young adult males between the ages of 20-35 years, use among teenagers also appears to be increasing rapidly. We have received calls from crack uers in at least 25 different states with most saying that the drug is "readily available" in their area. Only one year ago, not a single Hotline caller had mentioned crack. Similarly, over 75% of recent cocaine admissions to our inpatient and outpatient treatment programs at Regent Hospital and Stony Lodge Hospital have been for crack-related problems. Only nine months ago, not a single admission was for crack. Drug dealers prefer to sell crack rather than cocaine powder because of its higher profits, ease of handling, and also because the higher addiction potential of crack insures the dealer a more reliable clientele. Users prefer crack to powder because of its lower unit cost ($10-$20 for a vial of crack vs. $75-$100 for a gram of powder) and for its more potent, instantaneous euphoria or "rush".

The physical and psychological effects of smoking cocaine freebase differ in several important respects from those of snorting cocaine powder. Smoking cocaine is a very efficient and rapid drug delivery system. A single deep inhalation of the freebase smoke produces a sharp, rapid increase in the concentration of cocaine that gets into the bloodstream and the brain. Inhalations tend to be repeated as often as every three to five minutes during prolonged smoking "binges" that may extend over 1-3 days of continuous use until supplies of cocaine are depleted or the user collapses from exhaustion. The user may consume 10-30 grams or even several ounces of cocaine over the course of a typical binge. This pattern of use is extremely hazardous.

In smoking freebase cocaine there is substantial risk of toxic and overdose reactions such as brain seizures, heart attack and stroke as well as paranoid psychotic reactions leading to irrational, explosive behavior and violence. Significant lung damage and abnormalities have been documented in heavy freebase smokers which may persist long after cessation of the drug use. Chronic freebase smoking can also cause irritation and tissue damage to the user's eyes, lips, tongue, throat and pharynx. Many exhibit extreme hoarseness and a "raspy" voice for at least several days after use.

As compared to snorting cocaine, freebase smoking typically produces a more intense and more rapid euphoria, higher blood levels and brain concentrations of cocaine, a more powerful compulsion to return to the drug-induced state and thus a more rapid escalation to frequent and intensified usage patterns. Freebase smoking also causes a more intense and unpleasant cocaine "crash", and more serious medical and psychiatric consequences. Freebase smokers are more likely than snorters to require initial hospitalization in order to disrupt the pattern of compulsive use and to properly treat the more severe medical and psychiatric problems. Crack users require intensive follow-up care and may be expected to show higher relapse rates in early recovery. Outpatient treatment of the crack user requires daily counseling and a highly structured program including immediate family involvement and intensive planning of daily activities to avoid potential "triggers" of drug use.

ADOLESCENTS AND COCAINE

There continue to be dramatic increases in the numbers of adolescents abusing cocaine. Just since 1983, there has been a sevenfold increase in the number of teenagers (age 13-19) who call the 800-COCAINE National Helpline.

A survey of these teenage callers has provided some information about how their cocaine use is affecting them. Most teenage respondents in this survey were snorting cocaine, although 12% said they had switched to more intensified methods of use. Since the survey, however, "crack" or ready-to-smoke freebase "rocks" have become readily available to teens and the numbers of teenagers smoking freebase is thought to have sharply increased — particularly in urban areas.

A wide range of cocaine-related school, social, psychiatric and medical problems were reported by the adolescents surveyed. Seventy-five percent reported that their school performance had suffered considerably: 75% had missed days of school; 69% said grades had dropped significantly; 48% had experienced disciplinary problems due to drug-related changes in their mood or behavior; and 31% had been expelled for cocaine-related difficultues.

To support their escalating drug use, 44% of the teen respondents said they had sold drugs; 31% were stealing from family, friends or work; and 62% were using lunch or transportation money or income from a part-time job to buy drugs.

Among the most serious drug-related consequences reported by these teenage users were: cocaine-induced brain seizures with loss of consciousness (19%), cocaine-related automobile accidents (13%), suicide attempts (14%) and violent behavior (27%). Similar to adult users, common complaints included: insomnia, fatigue, depression, irritability, short-temper, paranoia, headaches, nasal and sinus problems, poor appetite, weight loss, memory and concentration problems, and heart palpitations. In most cases, loss of interest in non-drug-using friends, family activities and sports or hobbies were also reported.

It is important to note that among teenage Helpline callers, these serious consequences of cocaine use occurred more rapidly than among adult callers. The average teenager reported having used cocaine for the first time just one and one-half years prior to reaching this level of dysfunction, whereas the average adult caller reported using cocaine for four years before reaching a similar point of desperation.

Nearly every teenage subject said that the only limit on their cocaine use was money: if they had more money they would use more cocaine. The results of this survey show that adolescents do indeed have sufficient access to cocaine to become serious abusers and their vulnerability to the dependency-producing properties of the drug and to disrupted functioning may be even greater than that of adults.

Treatment Considerations:

First, because most adolescents in treatment are still living with their family (and even when living elsewhere are still very much affected by the family "system"), it is extremely important that the adolescent's family be involved in treatment. Without their participation, in fact, treatment is likely to be unsuccessful.

It is also wise for the clinician to obtain permission during the intake process to communicate with designated school personnel. Coordinating treatment with an assigned school counselor can provide the clinician with feedback about how the patient is functioning in school, and provide the patient with a greater sense of structure and consistency in his treatment.

Teenagers should be placed in a separate Cocaine Recovery Group with others of their own age. This, of course, promotes more rapid identification, and allows for the discussion of issues more relevant to teenagers. Also, the "positive" peer pressure that can develop in an adolescent recovery group to stop using cocaine can be as powerful and effective as teenage peer pressure to use.

Total abstinence from all mood-altering substances can, however, be an even more difficult issue for teens than for adults, and the clinician should remain aware of this. Many teenagers want to preserve their ability to use marijuana or to drink at least occasionally, and greatly fear the stigma they associate with remaining completely drug-free. Yet, the same poor prognosis exists for cocaine-abusing teens who continue to use any drugs.

Finally, the issue of driving while intoxicated with cocaine needs to be emphasized with adolescents, as their rate of cocaine-related accidents remains high. Combining cocaine with alcohol (stimulant with depressant) is very common among teen users and poses a particular danger when driving. Because cocaine's short-term stimulant effects temporarily mask the depressant effects of alcohol, the cocaine user is able to consume a large quantity of alcohol and initially not feel the intoxicating effects of the alcohol that might otherwise lead him to refrain from driving. When the cocaine wears off in only 20-30 minutes, the driver may suddenly become severely intoxicated or even stuperous from the alcohol with resulting gross and unexpected impairment of driving ability. Parents of adolescents in treatment need to be educated about this danger and helped to set clear limits about the use of a car if the adolescent continues to be a chemical abuser.

WOMEN AND COCAINE

Females age 18-34 comprise the fastest growing group of new drug users in the U.S., according to recent government surveys, and the drug many of these women are using is apparently cocaine. In 1985 nearly half the callers to the 800-COCAINE National Helpline were female, compared with one-third in 1983.

Reasons for this increase include the lowered cost of cocaine, more disposable income among females, greater availability through both the workplace and social situations, and the entry of more women into high-pressure jobs. The same appeal cocaine has to men in relieving fatigue and bolstering confidence applies, of course, to women. In addition, cocaine is often offered to women in social and sexual situations as a "gift" from cocaine-using men. Housewives also are attracted to cocaine as a way to relieve boredom and see themselves as participants in a popular trend. Finally, among women with eating disorders, the appetite-suppressing qualities of cocaine make it particularly attractive.

Treatment Considerations:

First, entering treatment may be more difficult for women than for men, given the additional stigma many experience. Our culture makes more allowances for men to "lose control" or be "wild" than for women. Thus, women who are seen as failing to perform their roles as "moral gatekeepers" in society are often judged more harshly than their male counterparts.

Women also tend to feel more guilt and humiliation about their drug abuse — and specifically about any sexual acting-out that they participated in while using cocaine. To help counter this greater resistance and embarrassment, clinicians should make special efforts to communicate a nonjudgmental attitude toward women in treatment.

Family members of women in treatment may react to the drug use with profound feelings of disappointment, anger and confusion. It is often hard for husbands and children of drug abusers in particular to view their wife or mother as someone in need of help and support since she may be thought of as the one in the family who is supposed to take care of others. It may be particularly important, then, to involve the family members of a female patient in the treatment process.

Cocaine use during pregnancy may adversely affect the development of the fetus, according to recent studies, and women in treatment need to be given information about this. Cocaine use causes irregular menstrual cycles in some women and occasionally female abusers have no menstruation at all.

Believing that they are unable to become pregnant, they may unwittingly subject the fetus to cocaine throughout its early development.

Among female substance abusers, problems in relationships with men appear to be a central concern and should be given careful consideration by the clinician. Often, a woman's cocaine use is closely connected with a particular relationship, so that stopping cocaine may also involve substantial additional feelings of loss.

Depression is also more commonly reported by women who abuse cocaine, as is sexual dysfunction and eating disorders. The clinician needs to remain particularly aware of these possibilities.

In addition to participation in a coed Cocaine Recovery Group, women in treatment may also benefit from a time-limited issue-oriented women's group. Here, participants often feel more comfortable discussing sexual experiences and problems resulting from cocaine use as well as issues related to relationships and identity.

If a female patient states a preference for a female counselor or therapist, this request should be met if possible. The very fact that a greater degree of comfort, rapport and trust is expected may contribute to greater ease in forming a therapeutic relationship. Cocaine abuse treatment programs should employ sufficient numbers of female counselors to meet this need.

SUMMARY

The truth is out about cocaine. No longer can it be regarded as a harmless "recreational" drug, providing instant euphoria and self-confidence with no price to pay. Nor can cocaine be dismissed as the "folly" of a rich and famous few — an indulgence made possible only by fabulous income and a penchant for excesses.

Today cocaine dependency is the fastest growing drug problem in our society. Cocaine is now cheaper, more readily available and used by a wider cross-section of people than ever before. Treatment of the casualties of this epidemic requires special attention.

We have attempted in this short space to provide guidelines and specific suggestions for treating the cocaine abuser. What we hope has been underscored is the fact that the drug cocaine has specific and unique features, namely its pharmacological effects on the brain's reward center, that can cause a particularly rapid and debilitating addiction. That addiction is characterized by drug cravings and urges that remain strong and unrelenting long into recovery.

It is these unique features of cocaine and cocaine abuse that dictate the need for specific guidelines in treating the cocaine abuser. Treatment programs of all kinds can be adapted to embrace these guidelines and effectively treat cocaine addicts. Each program and approach will be unique and hopefully responsive to the needs of its own particular patient group, but there should remain a certain common framework.

A clear and unwavering requirement of total abstinence from cocaine and all other mood-altering drugs should be the underpinning of any cocaine abuse treatment program. Without this "bottom line" requirement, there can be no effective treatment. Supervised urine testing is essential to document this abstinence, maintain the integrity of the program, and aid the patient in countering the strong drug urges and cravings with which he will undoubtedly struggle. It has also been our experience that the peer identification and support of a Cocaine Recovery Group is both beneficial and critical to patient abstinence.

Merely helping the patient to *become* abstinent, however, is never enough, and it is here that the most central element of long-term recovery must be applied — the teaching of relapse prevention techniques. For unless the predictable drug urges and cravings and the recurrent rationalization and denial characteristic of cocaine addiction are addressed, the patient will inevitably return to drug use and drop out of treatment. Getting a cocaine abuser "off" cocaine without teaching him how to *stay off* is the equivalent of detoxifying an alcoholic and then sending him off to work in a bar, or expecting a compulsive overeater to keep weight off after ending a "crash diet" when eating habits haven't changed. The point is that unless substantial changes are made in the way a cocaine abuser handles drug urges and cravings, and indeed in the very manner in which he conducts his life, there can be little hope for *long-term* rehabilitation. And in the end, if we don't help out patients along the road to lasting recovery but merely aid them in sporadic "clean-up" efforts, we may become more a part of the problem than the solution.

References

Gold, M.S. 800-COCAINE. New York: Bantam, 1984.

Gold, M.S., Washton, A.M., Dackis, C.A. Cocaine abuse: neurochemistry, phenomenology, and treatment. In: Kozel, N.J., Adams, E.H. (eds), Cocaine use in America: Epidemiologic and clinical perspectives. NIDA Research Monograph No. 61, DHHS pub. no. (ADM) 85-1414, Washington, D.C. Sup't of Docs, US Gov't Printing Office, 1985, pp. 130-150.

Marlatt, G.A., Gordon, J.R. Relapse prevention: Maintenance strategies in the treatment of addictive behaviors. New York: Guilford, 1985.

Stone, N., Fromme, M., Kagan, D. Cocaine: seduction and solution. New York: Clarkson N. Potter, 1984.

Verebey, K., Martin, D., Gold, M.S. Drug abuse: interpretation of laboratory tests. In: Gold, M.S., Pottash, A.C. (eds), Diagnostic and laboratory testing in psychiatry. New York: Plenum, pp. 155-167, 1986.

Washton, A.M. Cocaine abuse treatment. Psychiatry Letter, 1985; 3, 51-56.

Washton, A.M. Structured outpatient treatment of cocaine abuse. Advances in Alcohol and Substance Abuse, in press.

Washton, A.M. The "crack" epidemic. Written and oral testimony presented before the New York State Senate Committee on Investigations and Taxation. New York, N.Y., May 8, 1986.

Washton, A.M., Gold, M.S. Chronic cocaine abuse: evidence for adverse effects on health and functioning. Psychiatric Annals, 1984; 14, 733-743.

Washton, A.M., Gold, M.S. (eds.). Cocaine abuse: Recent trends and clinical perspectives. New York: Guilford, in press.

Washton, A.M., Gold, M.S., Pottash, A.C. Opiate and cocaine dependencies: techniques to help counter the rising tide. Postgraduate Medicine, 1985; 77, 293-300.

Washton, A.M., Hendrickson, E., Stone N. Clinical assessment of the cocaine abuser. In: Donovan, D., Marlatt, G.A. (eds), Assessment of addictive behaviors. New York: Guilford, in press.

Booklets Available From the American Council for Drug Education

Cocaine Today. Cohen, S. $2.50.

Cocaine: The Bottom Line. Cohen, S. $2.50.

Getting Tough on Gateway Drugs: A Guide for the Family. DuPont, R. L. $6.50.

A School Answers Back: Responding to Student Drug Use. Hawley, R. A. $5.00.

Marijuana Today: A Compilation of Medical Findings for the Layman. Russell, G. K. $3.00.

Marijuana Smoking and Its Effects on the Lungs. Tashkin, D. P. and Cohen, S. $2.50.

Marijuana and Reproduction. Smith, C. G. and Asch, R. H. $2.50.

Marijuana: The National Impact on Education. $2.50.

Marijuana and Alcohol. Cohen, S. and Lessin, P. J. $2.50.

Marijuana and Driving. Moskowitz, H. and Petersen, R. $2.50.

Treating the Marijuana-Dependent Person. de Silva, R. and DuPont, R. L. (Eds.) $3.00.

The Marijuana Controversy: Definition, Research Perspective and Therapeutic Claims. Turner, C. E. $2.50.

Urine Testing for Marijuana Use: Implications for a Variety of Settings. Blasinsky, M. and Russell, G. K. (Eds.) $2.50.

A Pediatrician's View of Marijuana. Lanter, I. and Barth, R. $2.50.

Therapeutic Potential of Marijuana's Components. Cohen, S. and Andrysiak, T. $2.50.

When ordering, enclose check payable to **ACDE**. Please add 10% of total order to cover the cost of postage and handling.

Free catalog on additional materials and films available upon written request.